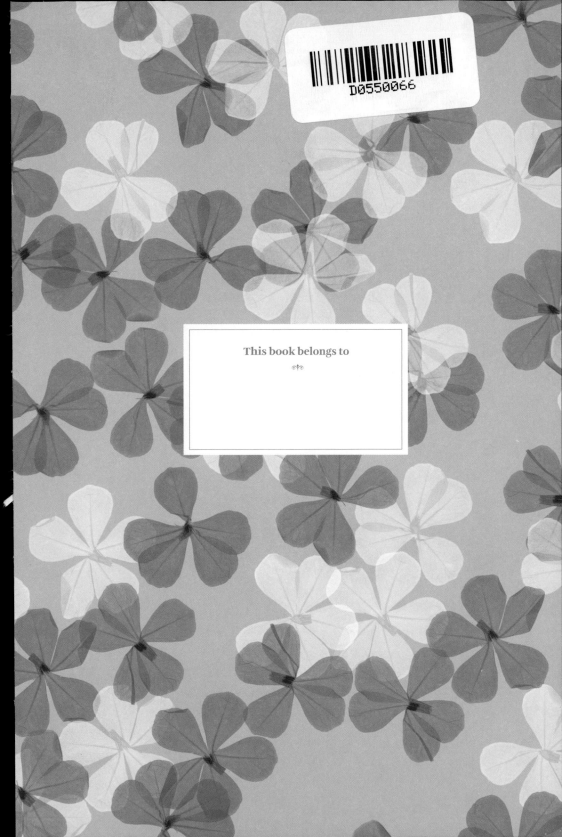

This book belongs to

❦

*I dedicate this book to my
beautiful Justin, who reminds
me to always follow my heart*

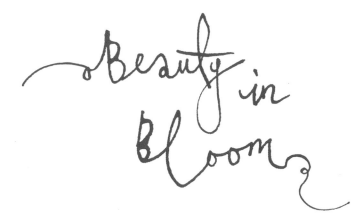

Beauty in Bloom

A collection of
beautiful inspirations

Natalie Bloom and
Emma-Charlotte Bangay

❦

Illustrations by
Rebecca Wetzler

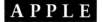

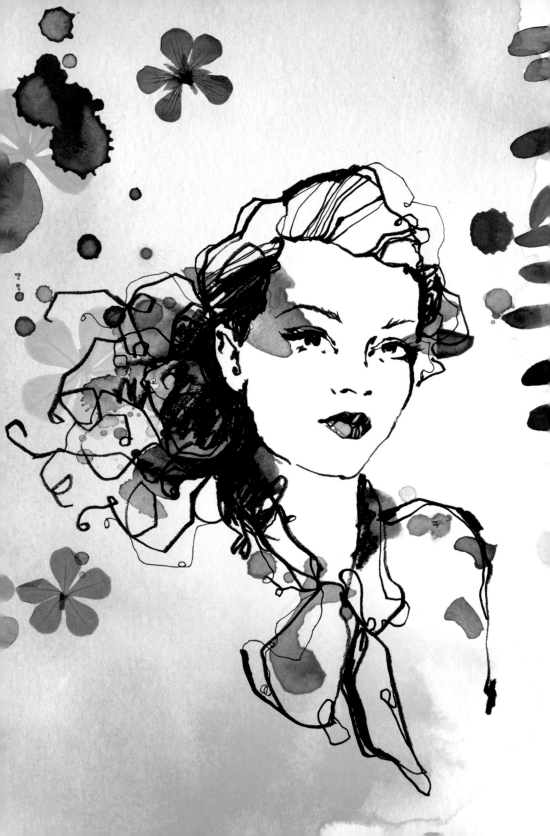

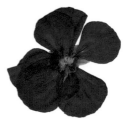

Introduction

❀

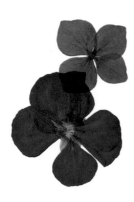

Beauty in Bloom

Introduction

❦

Beauty in Bloom is a scrapbook of all the things that make my heart skip a beat, make me feel good, and have excited, invigorated and spurred me on in both my business and personal life.

With my business ever expanding and my children taking me on dizzying daily adventures, I have little time to write a shopping list let alone a book. So when the idea for *Beauty in Bloom* came along and began to set off the inspiration bells in me, my head told me not to take on the project, but my heart kept tapping away at the keys, unveiling all that I love, find inspiring and feel is truly beautiful.

To me, beauty is a collaboration of many elements. Makeup is definitely a powerful factor, but having a positive attitude, great personal style, nurturing your body and surrounding yourself with the things you love go hand in hand with creating your own beauty.

Beauty in Bloom is my way of sharing and celebrating all the beautiful things that have touched my heart. I hope it encourages you to pursue your passion, introduces a fresh vision to your eyes and brings a secret smile to your lips.

Natalie Bloom
Founder, Bloom Cosmetics

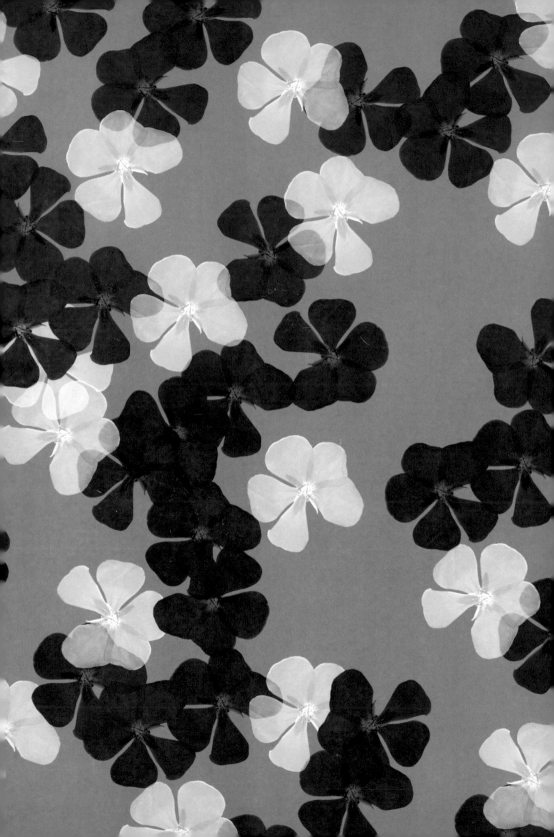

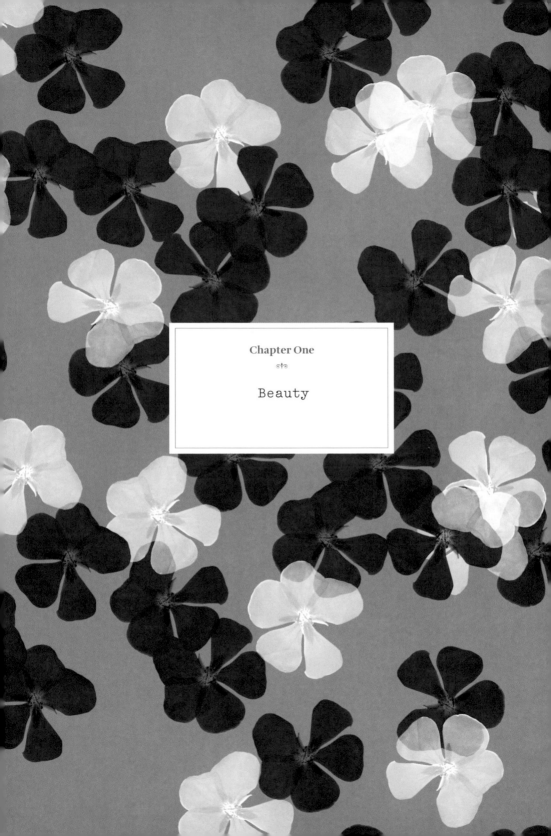

Chapter One

⚬❦⚬

Beauty

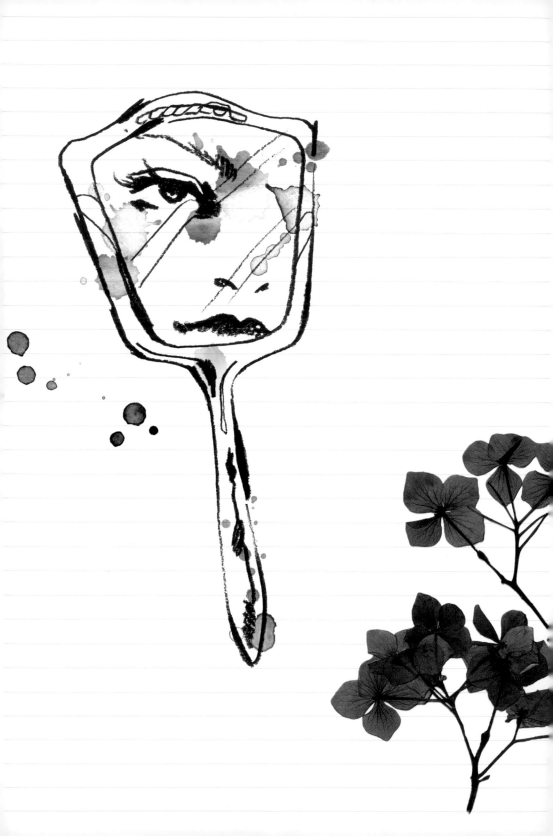

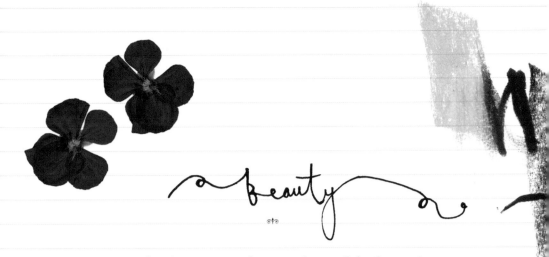

beauty

In today's super-charged world, there is a certain romance and ritual to applying makeup. It is often one of the few moments when you can enjoy some time to yourself, and even the simplest sweep of mascara or lip gloss can literally change the colour of your day.

Smile when you look in the mirror, see the positives in the signs of time on your face, and show it the respect and daily TLC it deserves.

Some basic everyday care and shelter from the sun are simple steps towards keeping your skin looking its very best, no matter what your age.

What's not to love about makeup?

Makeup seduced me long ago. As a young girl, I spent
hours experimenting and playing with the colours and
textures of cosmetics.

And to this day, it still delivers that little bit of magic.
No matter where I am, I will always apply makeup.

When I think back, I can trace this love affair with all things
beauty back to my grandmother and mother. Thanks to
them, makeup is in my make-up.

I remember sitting in my grandmother's boudoir,
rummaging through her collection of treasured Chanel
lipsticks, eye shadows and nail polishes and being
enchanted by the shades, scents and possibilities they
represented. I still cherish her vintage lipstick cases with
the half-used lipstick forever marked with her lips.

My mother, too, would never leave the house without
impeccable makeup. I recall watching her with fascination
as she applied it meticulously before going out. Often
she would let me play with the fabulous colours and creams
scattered across her beauty cabinet. It was every little
girl's dream.

Cherish the ritual of applying makeup. No matter how
much or little time you have, relish that precious moment
in your day. Fall head over heels for colour, feel the silken
textures and be intoxicated by how cosmetics can make
you look and feel.

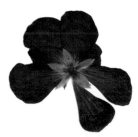

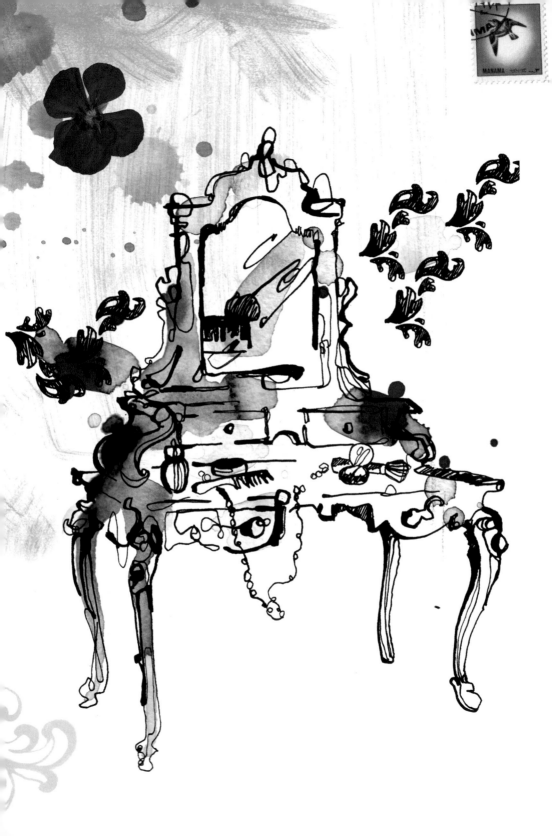

Beauty secrets

There are no rules with makeup. It's about fun, creativity and experimentation.

Throughout history, makeup has been used as a tool of expression and enhancement of a character, from a Geisha's fragile face to tough tribal markings or Cleopatra's kohl-rimmed eyes.

But makeup is not a mask. It is intended to enhance your eyes, lips and cheeks, not conceal the real you! If you're like me, your everyday application calls for a few simple ideas. Here are some I live by.

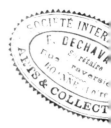

Primer

Primer creates an ideal canvas for your makeup.
Just as you would apply a base coat of paint to your
house, primer is an essential step to even out your
skin tone prior to putting on makeup. A relatively
new kid on the beauty block, this must-have tool
is rapidly becoming indispensable.

Foundation

Take baby steps with foundation, building up
gradually as you go. Make sure you're using a
consistency and colour that suits.

As a general rule:
Liquid foundations are lovely for every day, and
work well on drier skins.

·

Stick foundations get a ten out of ten for great
convenience and coverage. They also work well to
conceal dark circles under eyes and uneven tone
around the nose.

·

Pure mineral powder foundations are especially
kind on sensitive skins. Additive free, pure mineral
makeup delivers a luminous sheen in seconds.

·

Pressed powder is best for high coverage and
oilier complexions.

To get your foundation-shade-to-skin match right,
test foundations on the jawline (not your hand)
and always do so in natural daylight.

Illuminiser

Illuminisers are my favourite way to brighten the skin and add a translucent sheen. Apply directly to the areas that light naturally hits for added glow, or try mixing a bit with your favourite liquid foundation or moisturiser for a more subtle effect.

Brushes

When it comes to your beauty budget, brushes are the best place to splurge. The difference between using a good-quality makeup brush and a cheaper version is like cashmere to cotton. Choose your brush to fit the purpose: goat, squirrel and pony-haired brushes are soft and kind when applying powder foundation, powder eye shadows or cheek colour. On the other hand, synthetic fibres work wonders for liquid foundations or more precise lines around the brows and eye line.

Blending

Blend, blend, blend! The biggest beauty faux pas is failing to blend away any edges and lines on all kinds of makeup: concealer, blush, bronzer, eye shadow, lip liner and, most commonly, foundation.

Smoothing your foundation from the jawline down towards the neck until it disappears only takes a few seconds, so be sure to do it! Blending should be your basic makeup mantra, so whether you use a brush, your fingertips or a sponge, this is one beauty area where the line is always best blurred.

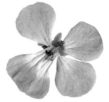
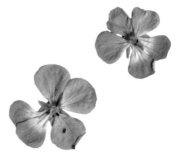

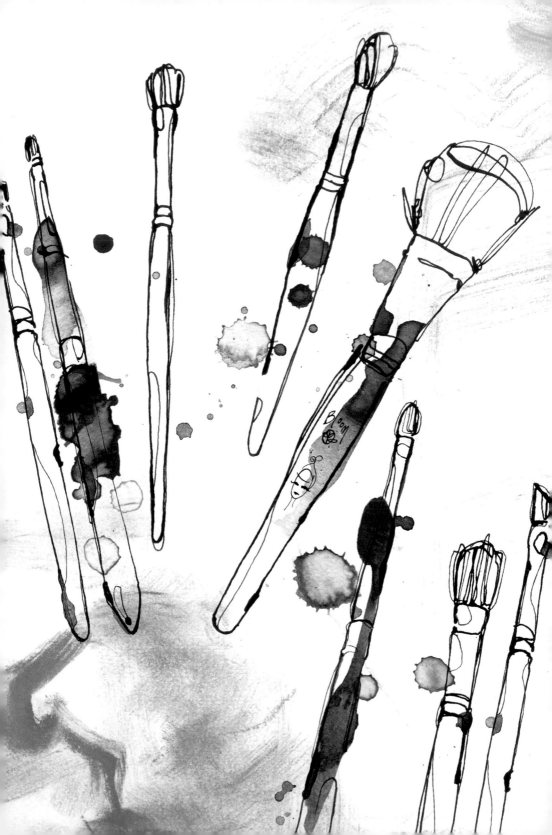

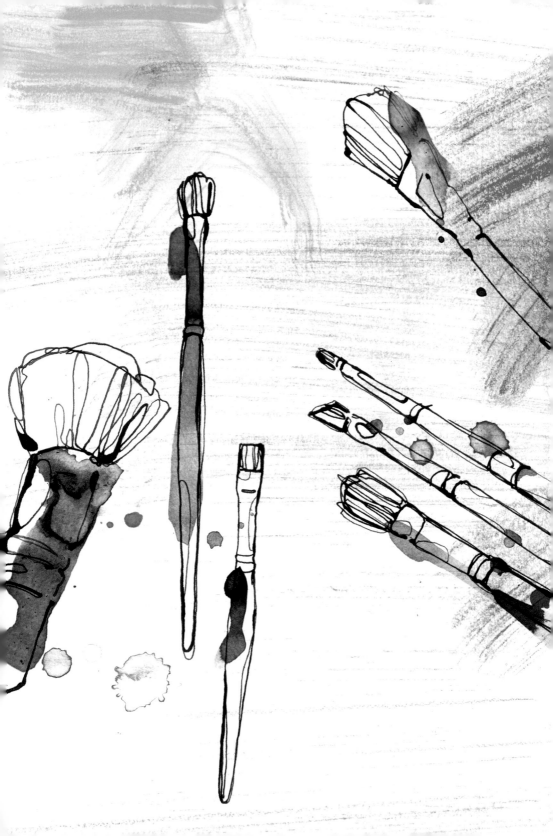

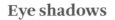

Eye shadows

Eye shadow is one of the bravest and boldest cosmetics for changing your look, and the options are endless.

Begin by applying a light base colour all over the eye, extending across the eyelid and up to the brow. Then use a darker shade to contour along the socket crease and, finally, apply the darkest colour along the lash line, from inner-eye to outer edge.

Remember, though, rules are meant to be broken! So don't be afraid to take yourself out of your cosmetic comfort zone and dabble in a touch of vibrant colour. Introduce a bright, brave shade along the lash line or over the entire eyelid on those days you want to live bright not bland.

Mascara

Mascara is the magic wand of makeup. Sure you can pinch your cheeks and lick your lips, but there is nothing more charming than fluttery, flirty, come-hither lashes to bat at whoever is looking your way.

Begin applying mascara by hugging the lash line then wiggle the wand out to the tips, layering for a more dramatic effect. Remember not to pump the wand up and down in the bottle otherwise air gets in and will dry the mascara out. Replace your mascara every six months to ensure you are getting a fresh coat of colour with each application.

Eyelash curlers

Armed with an eyelash curler? Then the magic of a butterfly kiss is forever within your reach.

To really lash out, curl eyelashes before applying your mascara. I get the best results by gently heating my aluminium eyelash curler with a hair dryer for a few seconds before placing the curler as close to the base of lashes as possible. Squeeze for 10 seconds and let go. Voilà!

full and flirty

Little tip

If you haven't been blessed with naturally long lashes, all is not lost. You can create the illusion of fuller lashes by simply applying eyeliner to the inside upper rim of the eye. For added oomph, add a few short individual false lash pieces to the outer corners of eyelashes.

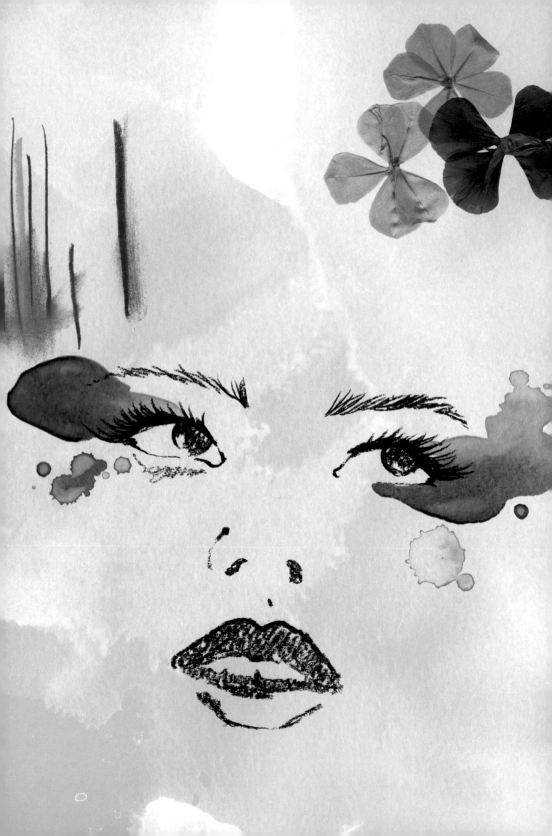

'The best colour in the whole world is the one that looks good on you.'

Coco Chanel

Nail polish

From sheer seashell pink to tangy orange or
super pink, I'm mad for nail polish. Maybe it's
hereditary—my grandmother always had glossy
red nails! While I rarely have time for a manicure,
a quick lick of lacquer is my instant pick-me-up.
It's my chocolate of fashion.

It may seem obvious, but my golden rule for nail
polish is that no matter how short on time I am,
two thin coats are always better than one thick
coat. Give each layer 60 seconds to dry and you'll
find that your polish will dry faster and last longer.

Brows

Thick and dramatic or arched and elegant; brows
frame the eyes. Keeping them well groomed is one
of the easiest ways to really make a difference to
the way you look. Neat, well-shaped brows add an
element of grace even if you are makeup-free. So
get a professional shape initially to ensure you are
on the right track, and from there you should be
able to tweak your shape with tweezing.

When shading in brows, use an eyebrow pencil
or a powder applied with a brush. Simply dip
the brush in the product and apply gently in soft
upward strokes rather than drawing a hard line.
Match your brow colour to the natural colour of
your hair and groom with a brow gel after shading.

Cream blush

Cream blush is the best when you're in a rush because it can be applied with the fingertips and it adds a flattering flush in a flash. But remember, whether you're happy, sad or simply indifferent, smiling is compulsory when applying blush to the apples of your cheeks as this cleverly indicates the natural rise of your cheekbone, pinpointing the area where you naturally blush.

Lip gloss

Yes, I am addicted to lip gloss! For me, lip gloss
is the holy grail of cosmetics. I can literally apply
it without a mirror and it gives me an instant
beauty boost.

I keep one (or three) stashed in my glove box,
handbag, work drawer and bathroom cabinet
for easy, anywhere application.

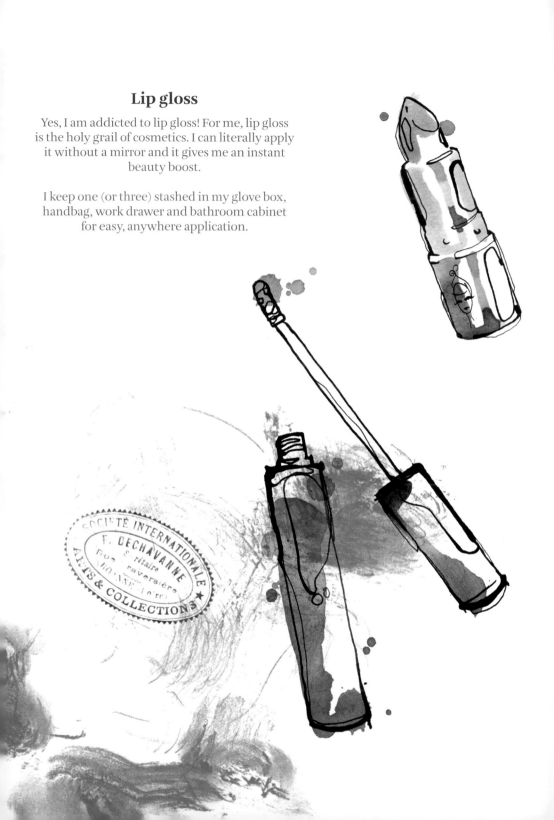

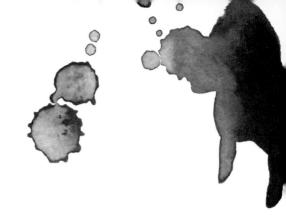

Lipstick

If gloss is not your go, opt for the classic allure of lipstick.

The quintessential cosmetic, lipstick is perennially pretty for day or night and has made its mark on several icons throughout history; from Marilyn Monroe to Dita Von Teese, Joan Crawford to Rita Hayworth, lipstick spells glamour.

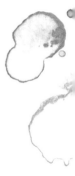

Lipstick has crossed the great divide between fashion and beauty, making it as memorable a style statement as a fabulous pair of shoes or a chic clutch.

Although its status became established decades ago, lipstick consistencies have improved over time. Lipsticks are now smooth, hydrating and long-lasting on the lips, while offering deep or subtle colour.

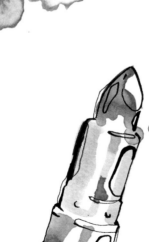

'The act of removing a lipstick's top
and then turning the bottom, letting the
lipstick appear and go straight to kiss
the lips in waiting. Changing one's
facial expression—a bit like putting the
light on in a dark room.'

Mirka Mora
Love and Clutter

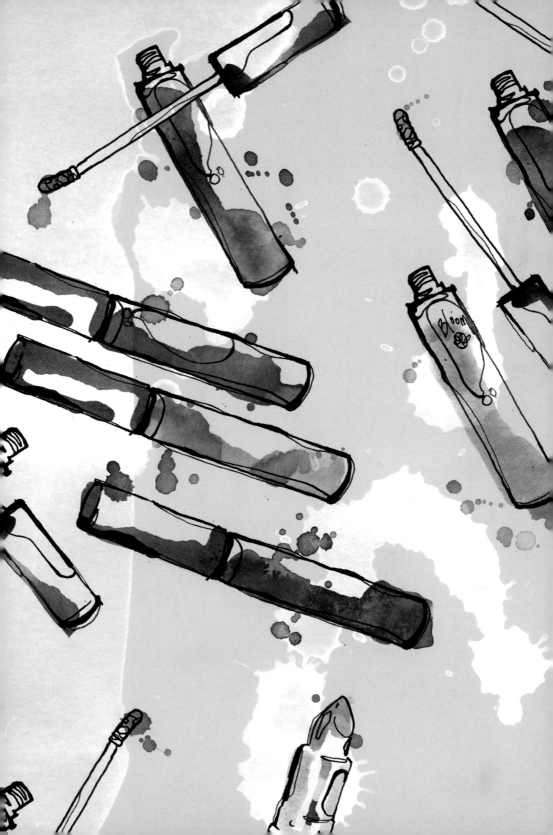

Textures

Cosmetics are to the face what paint is to a canvas. As the colours available have reached a kaleidoscopic climax, so too have textures blossomed to suit every tone, every type, every day. Ebb and flow through the options, but remember your skin can change with the seasons, your mood and your age, so keep an eye on your perfect match!

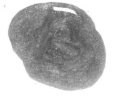

Sheer
Sheer makeup drops colour pigment down a gear, giving an almost 'no makeup' effect. It suits most skin tones with its barely-there coverage and it's hard to make a mistake with sheer colour.

Shimmer
Shimmer products contain light-reflecting properties that have a flattering effect on skin. Only apply where light naturally hits your face, highlighting the parts of your face you want accentuated.

Matte

Welcome matte textures when you want to keep a glow at bay. Perfect for oily complexions, matte shades are usually denser in colour than their shimmery, sheer siblings and give more coverage for longer-lasting results.

Gloss

There's no denying, gloss screams fun! Flirty! GLAMOUR! High-gloss textures are the best for lips, but you can be adventurous and also use them lightly across eyelids and cheeks to give a natural sheen.

Satin

A satin finish is halfway between gloss and matte. It delivers what it promises: a satiny, smooth, even, subtle finish. Colour is flat, but not matte.

Everyday care

You and your skin are younger now than you will ever be again, so enjoy the way you look today and take time to look after your most important asset.

For most of us flawless skin may be a fantasy, but with a little care it can actually become fact. The golden rule is that skin should be prepped and polished with three simple steps: cleansing, exfoliating and moisturising.

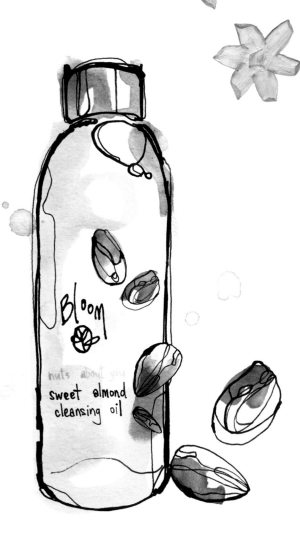

Bloom

nuts about you

sweet almond cleansing oil

Cleansing

It may sound strange, but cleansing oil is a great way to literally dissolve makeup without the need to scrub and tug at skin. Before you reject this option, exclaiming that your skin is already oily, relax. There is actually 'good oil' within the beauty world.

Cleansing with specially formulated oil won't necessarily make acne-prone or naturally oily skins break out. In fact, by stripping natural oils away with, say, a foaming cleanser, you are actually activating an SOS within the skin, tricking it into producing more oil. So give cleansing oil a go for a gentle, effective way to remove makeup and cleanse skin. I swear you'll be hooked!

Exfoliating

Exfoliating every other day is essential to get the most from moisturising your skin. It's the only way to get rid of dead skin cells and that nasty grit and grime build-up, leaving skin fresh and ready to soak up the benefits of hydration.

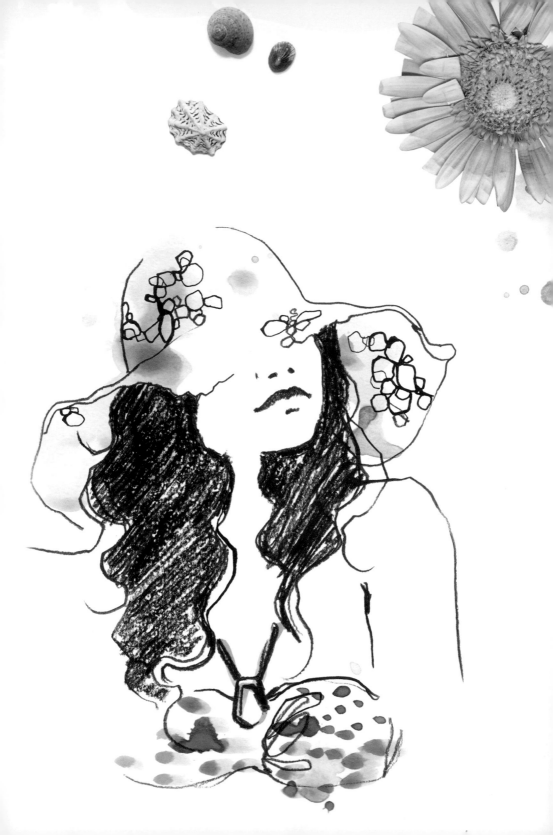

Moisturising

Creams, lotions and potions are key to locking moisture into your skin. This works wonders for temporarily plumping fine lines and smoothing dry patches, leaving skin to appear hydrated, fresher and more youthful.

In terms of turning back the clock, I believe prevention is better than cure. You know the drill: don't smoke, drink less alcohol, do exercise, eat well, sleep well and of course drink plenty of water. It may sound tired, but there is no denying, it's tried, tested and true. Not for a second do I think that beauty creams can erase wrinkles, but I do believe the ritual of applying them can nourish skin and give a more youthful appearance.

Unfortunately, our love affair with the sun means that most of us have spent the halcyon days of our youth catching some rays in nothing more than a crochet bikini and coconut oil, and only now are we paying the price. Although vitamin D from the sun has its essential benefits, the sun can wreak havoc on the skin, resulting in lines, wrinkles and pigmentation damage. Therefore, the only true anti-ageing product on the market is sunscreen. Take refuge in it—and shade—this summer. Your skin will thank you for it.

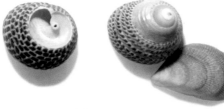

I have always believed in taking a natural approach to skincare. I believe products that are naturally scented with essential oils and jam-packed with botanical extracts make you and your skin feel more uplifted—not just your complexion. To me, skincare should also be a sensory experience. It makes sense to use some of the gifts that Mother Nature has given us. Believe me, I would love to sell an avocado in a jar. Or a tube of honey and egg yolk hair mask.

When you have only two pennies left in the world, buy a loaf of bread with one, and a lily with the other.

Chinese Proverb

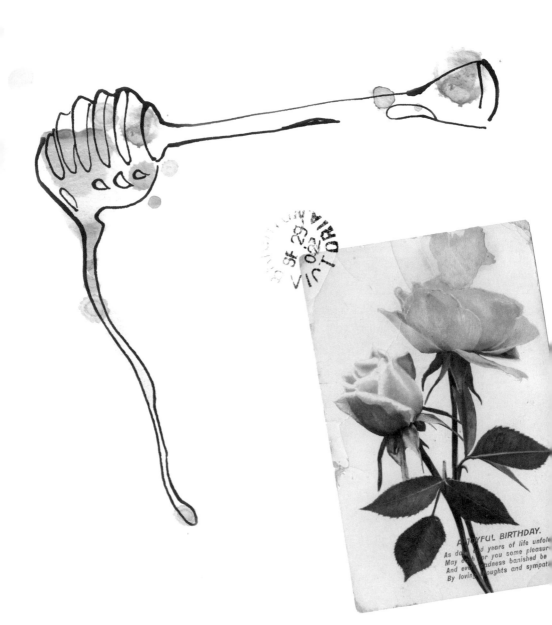

A JOYFUL BIRTHDAY.

As days and years of life unfold
May each for you some pleasure
And every sadness banished be
By loving thoughts and sympath

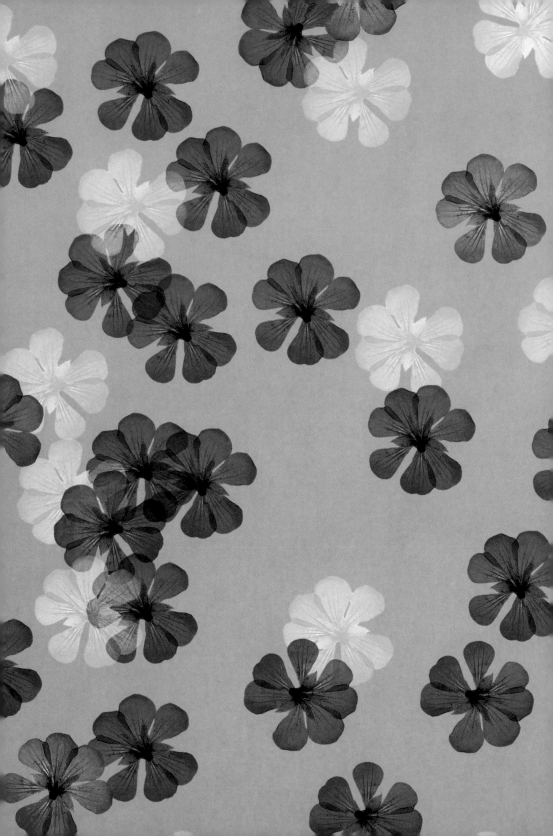

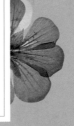

Chapter Two

❖

```
Indefinable Beauty
```

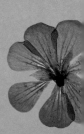

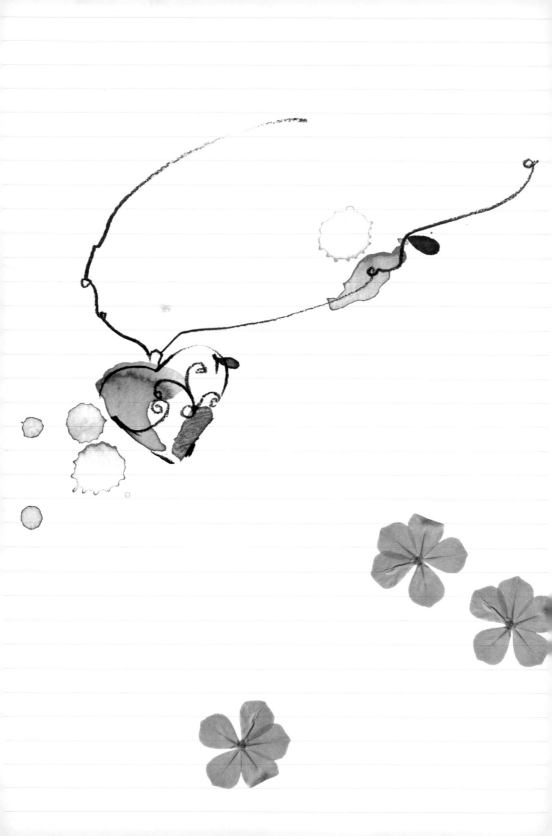

Undefinable Beauty

No matter what cosmetic concoction you opt for, how you feel inside is written all over your face. There are no quick fixes and expert tricks when it comes to feeling beautiful, but embracing the everyday with open arms and an open heart can make all the difference.

Whether it's an innate sense of style, a driving passion or just a positive attitude, these intangible elements influence our beauty. So too does the way we nurture our bodies and look after ourselves.

Beauty inside and out

True beauty is indefinable. It isn't something you can buy or apply.

```
'Beauty is not in the face;
beauty is a light in the heart.'

           Kahlil Gibran
```

To me, a beautiful person is someone who is genuinely passionate with a lovely spark in their eyes, a huge smile on their face or has an intelligence or curiosity.

I am drawn to people who exude a positive attitude and their own sense of personal style. People who embrace their quirks, both inside and out, are beautiful. Not in a perfect, unattainable kind of way, but in a real sense.

Think about all the beautiful, stylish women you know. What do they have in common? The common thread is usually confidence, graceful style, passion or a unique twist in their approach to life. After all, nothing radiates more beautifully than a woman who is comfortable in her own skin.

I believe the new criteria for beauty should be character, wisdom and individuality.

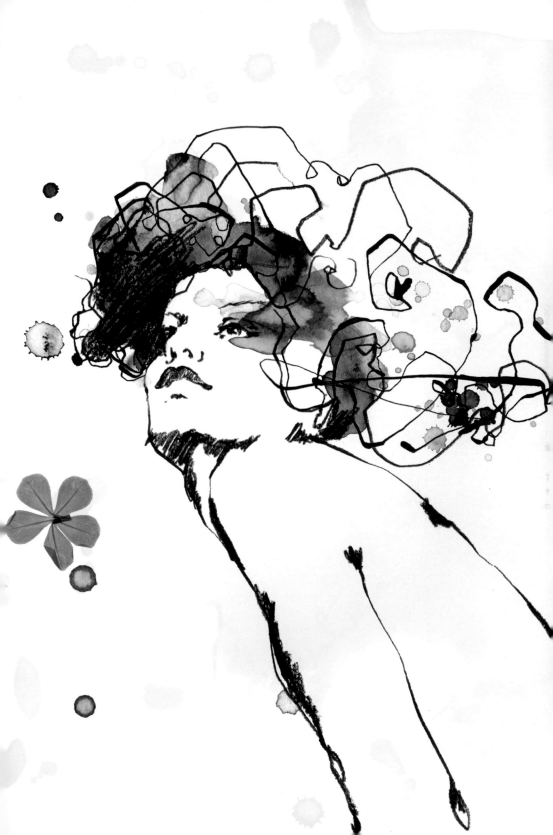

Style

There is nothing more captivating than someone who dresses with confidence and isn't a slave to fashion yet has a strong sense of what works for her and makes her feel comfortable.

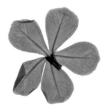

'Fashions fade,
style is eternal.'

Yves Saint Laurent

I love a woman who mixes designer brands
with vintage pieces and the odd chain-store gem.
In fashion, design and beyond we are incessantly
raiding the past, searching every nook and cranny
for the indescribable appeal of rare finds.
Scouring markets, vintage stores, country towns,
eBay ... anywhere we may be able to uncover
a hidden treasure.

The past is an endless source of ideas in my life,
work and style. Inspiration from yesteryear can
take many forms: a movie, a book, a piece of art
and even furniture.

I love to indulge in things that have a sense of
modern nostalgia and carry the meaning of the
past in a fast-moving present.

These are a couple of little essentials for everyday elegance.

Hankies are just so charming. I love their poetry and femininity. Always scent your hankies with perfume.

·

Beautiful stationery is so important. Forget longwinded, impersonal emails and relish in the charm of writing a sweet note on elegant stationery.

·

Good-quality, gorgeous **hosiery** is a symbol of style and elegance.

·

Lush **luxury soap** is such a simple indulgence. Invest in the best because life is too short for supermarket soap. Try storing soap in your top drawer to scent your lingerie.

Style is not just how you coordinate your clothes, the height of your heels, the hue of your hair or the brand of your handbag. It's how you walk, talk, carry a conversation and carry yourself. There is no paint-by-numbers formula to personal style, just one simple rule: stay true to yourself and don't overwork it. Style should be effortless and a relaxed, natural, easy breed of chic.

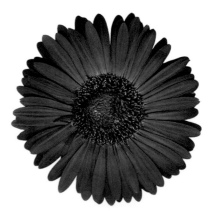

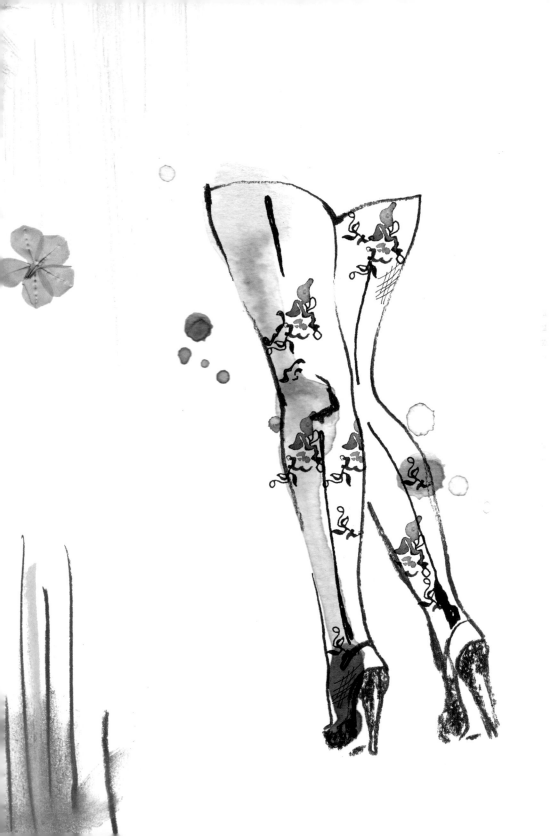

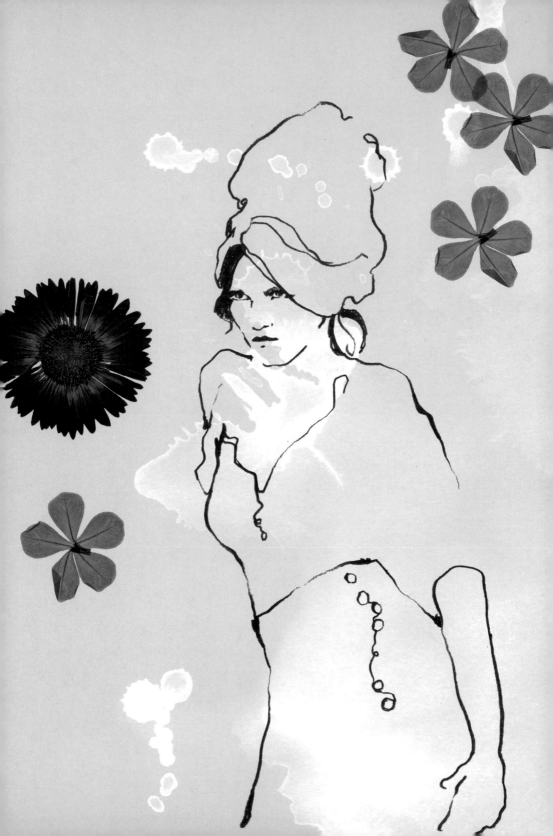

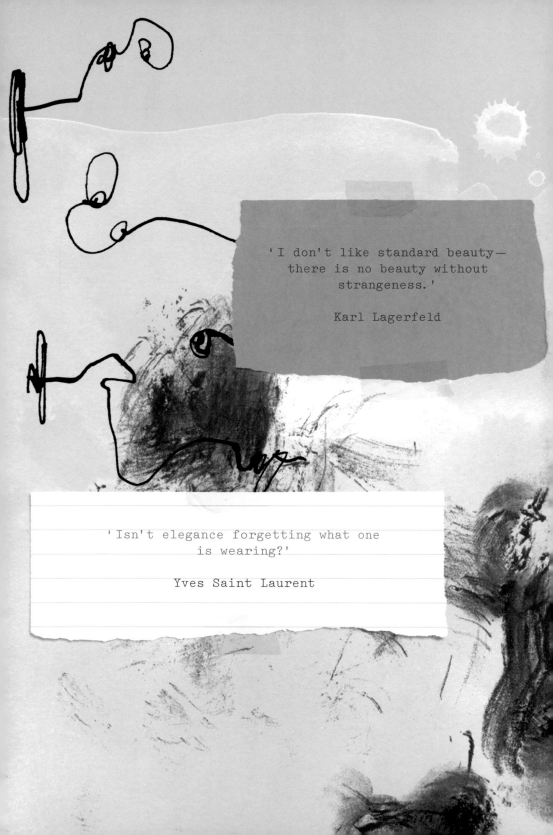

'I don't like standard beauty—
there is no beauty without
strangeness.'

Karl Lagerfeld

'Isn't elegance forgetting what one
is wearing?'

Yves Saint Laurent

An A–Z to inspire a positive attitude

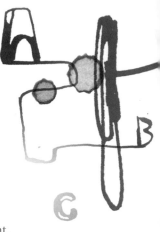

A
Attitude: a positive attitude is our inner light.
Turn it on and let it shine bright.

B
Believe in yourself in order for others to do
the same.

C
Charm your way out of anything!
It's a girl's 'get out of jail free' card.

D
Dream big.

E
Eclectic: mix and match to suit your mood;
don't follow one system of style.

F
Femininity is every woman's gift.
It's priceless and timeless.

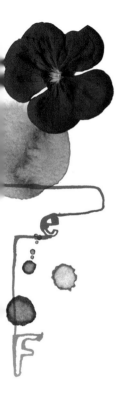

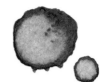

G

Glamour: an elegant pair of earrings,
a deeper shade of lipstick or a perfect
manicure.

H

Heart: never do something if your heart
is not in it.

I

Integrity: whatever you do, do it
with integrity.

J

Joie de vivre! The joy of life transcends
any language.

K

Kindness: make acts of kindness
regular rather than random.

L

Laughter is contagious. Pass it on!

M

Melbourne means home to me.
Love where you live.

N

New: always try something new.

O

Openness: keep an open mind and nurture
an open heart.

P

Poise and posture are essential in order to
walk tall through life.

Q

Quirkiness: add a dash of the unpredictable
into your day.

R

Respect your own decisions.

S

Spirit: your spirit is the engine room of
your life. Keep it stoked and enthusiastic.

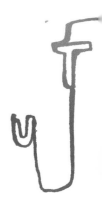

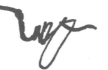

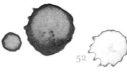

T
Touch should never be underestimated.
A hand to hold, a shoulder to cry on ...

U
Uniqueness is the difference between getting lost
in the crowd and standing out on your own.

V
Vision means seeing things not just for what they
are now, but what they can be in the future.

W
World: do your little bit to make a big difference.

X
X marks the spot. Put your stamp on something so
that it lingers on when you are long gone.

Y
You are only worth as much as you invest in
yourself. Love yourself. Be kind to yourself.
Appreciate yourself.

Z
Zest: *'Zest is the secret of all beauty.*
There is no beauty that is attractive without zest.'
Christian Dior

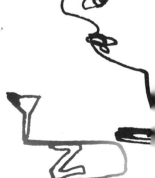

'For beautiful eyes, look for good in others, for beautiful lips, speak only words of kindness; and for poise, walk with the knowledge that you are never alone.'

Audrey Hepburn

'You can take no credit for beauty at sixteen. But if you are beautiful at sixty, it will be your soul's own doing.'

Marie Stopes

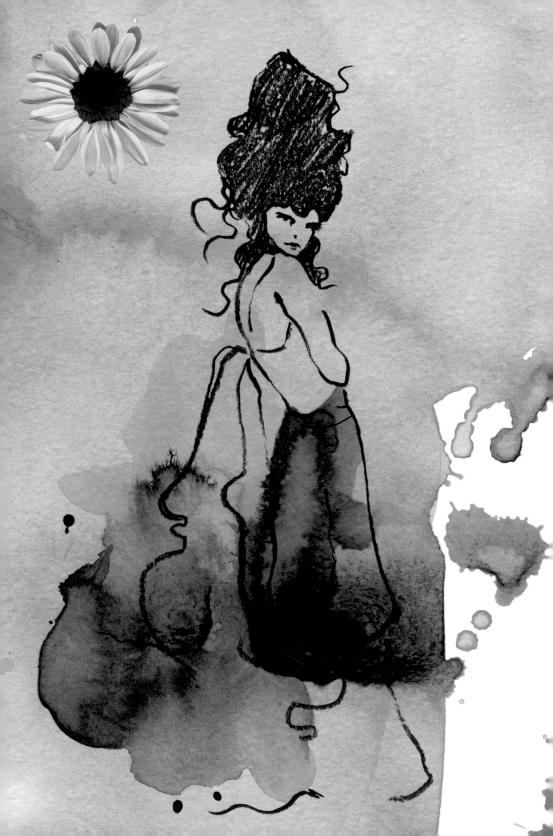

Beauty from nature

I believe in drawing upon the power of nature and its ingredients to nurture the body. It's a philosophy I live by and a core element of everything we do at Bloom. It's all about getting back to basics and letting nature be your beauty elixir.

Replenish your skin with water, cleanse your lungs with fresh air and nourish your mind and body with wholesome food and home-grown herbs. Limit sun exposure instead of looking for a miracle cream and draw on natural alternatives to make you feel as beautiful as life intended.

Long before they made the transition from hippie to hip, I have had a fierce interest in essential oils. Highly concentrated oils extracted from plants, fruits, flowers and herbs are definitely the better option compared to synthetic fragrances.

While synthetic fragrances are manufactured in the controlled atmosphere of a laboratory, essential oils are volatile—often depending on the elements. Consider this: 1000 kg of jasmine flowers yield approximately 1 kg of liquid concentrate. Get the picture?

Regardless, what could be more divine than using creams and lotions in the knowledge that the fragrance is all natural? You are instantly seduced by not only the nourishment but the sensory experience.

At home, try adding a drop of essential oil, or a blend of a few oils, to a bath, or mix a few drops into some olive oil and use as a body oil.

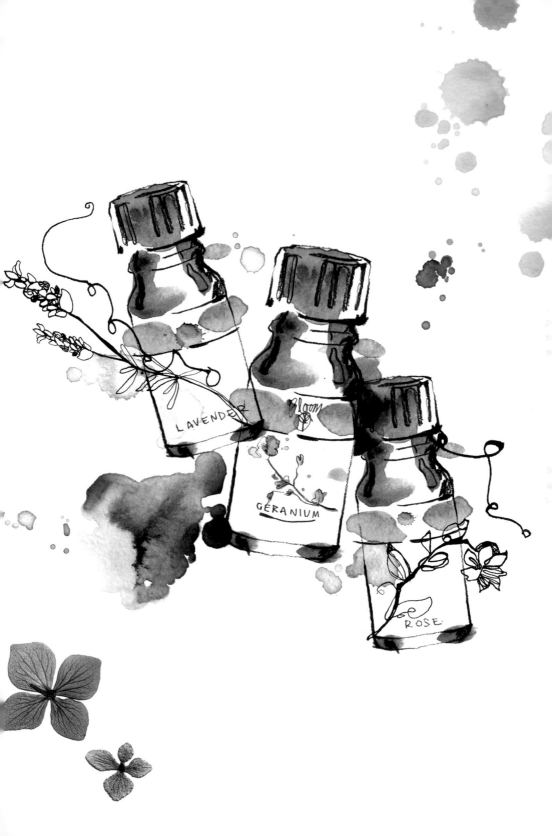

Herbs

A herb garden is your own little patch to nurture nature. No matter how humble your home, a herb garden only takes up the tiniest corner of the earth or a couple of terracotta pots to flourish.

Herbs are the quintessential plant—they look gorgeous, smell even better and do you the world of good. Pick from your own garden and add a dash to a dish, a touch in tea or a sprinkle to a stew. The personal touch to your cooking is worth the effort.

I particularly love it when my kids appreciate the joy of what the garden has to offer. When they pick some mint, parsley, basil, rosemary or dill for dinner they get such delight out of it and the dishes taste that little bit more delicious!

I love ...
Rosemary on potatoes
Mint in tea
Lemon verbena in water
Chopped continental parsley in soup
Basil on salad
Lavender by your pillow
Dill on fish

H₂O

Being hydrated means being healthy.
And it's simple to do. You don't have to eliminate
the lattes completely, but try kick-starting your
day with a glass of warm boiled water and a slice
of lemon. This will wake up the liver and rouse
complexion correction.

During the day, hit the bottle by stashing a 1.5
litre water jug at your desk, making sure you drink
it all before the day is done. Your skin will look
brighter, more revitalised and fresher.

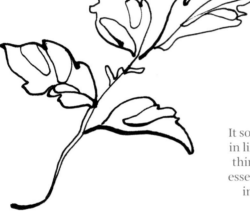

Time out

It sounds ridiculous, but as with many things
in life, we forget to take time to do the simple
things. Remembering to breathe properly is
essential. Drawing in deep, long breaths right
into the belly every now and again has a
calming effect.

For me the simplest thing to remember
when I am stressed is to take a deep breath
and move forward.

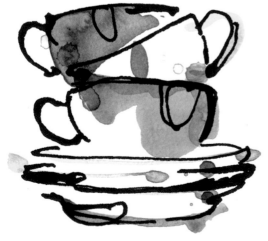

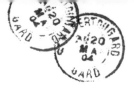

Food for thought

The foods you eat shouldn't be dictated by whether they will make you fat or thin, but by the enjoyment and goodness you can get out of each bite.

I always try to eat produce that is in season. When it comes down to it, if it's recently fallen from a tree or grown from the ground, I know it's better for me and my family.

I love the textures, aromas and colours of fresh ingredients. Eating a rainbow can fill you with so much goodness: the deep red of beetroot, the sunshine within an orange, the lush green of vegetables …

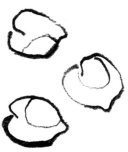

Ingredients I love to use in cooking:
chickpeas
quinoa
adzuki beans
kombu
umeboshi plums
nori
shiitake mushrooms
buckwheat noodles
tofu
tempeh
seeds
beetroot

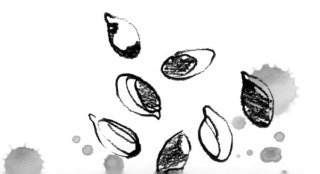

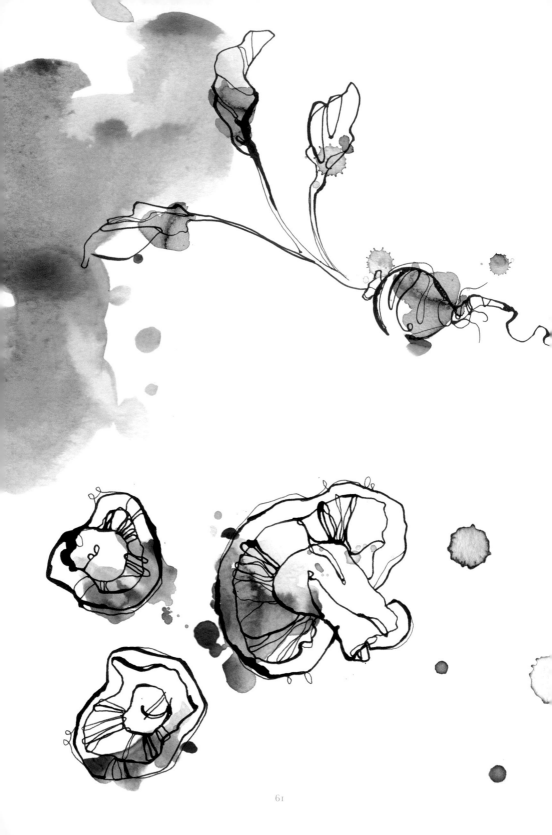

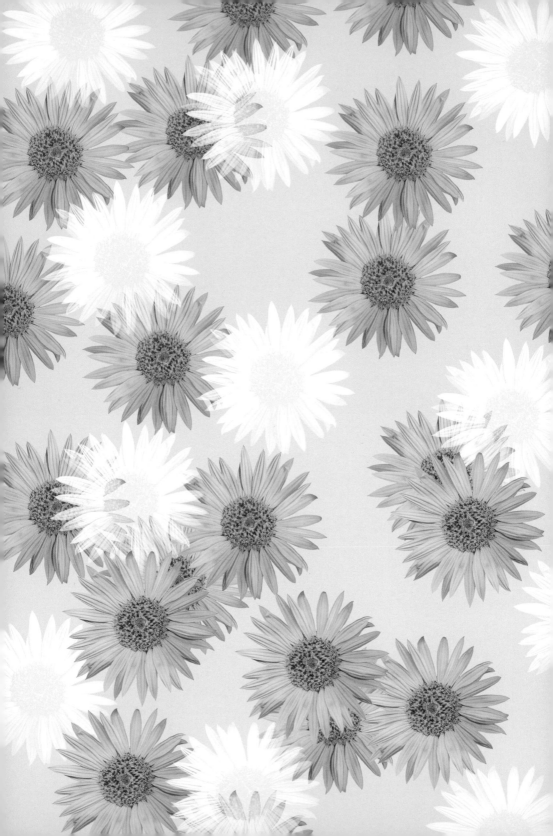

Chapter Three

❦

Beautiful to me

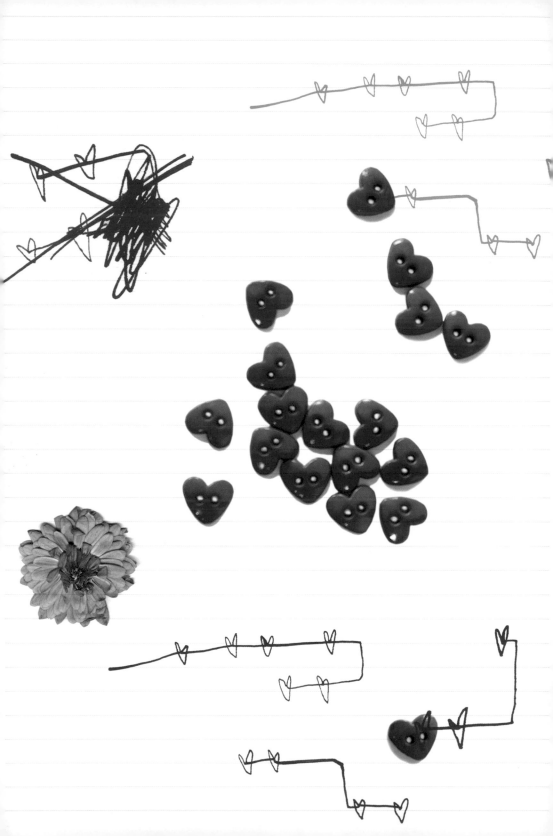

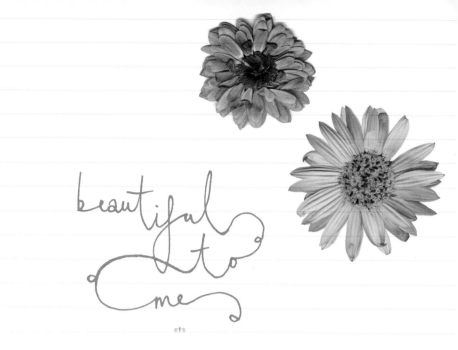

beautiful to me

> *There are many things in life that will catch your eye, but only a few will catch your heart ... pursue those.*
> Michael Nolan

If something touches your heart, hold it close to you. Finding such a gift isn't a one-time journey. Relish the constant quest towards feeling, collecting and creating what you love.

Surround yourself with what you love

Spontaneous inspiration when you least expect it can elevate you to do amazing things. I am living proof of that. I started Bloom simply because I love design and packaging. I responded to a moment of inspiration and now years later it has evolved into a business and rewarding vocation.

'The best and most beautiful things in the world cannot be seen or even touched. They must be felt with the heart.'

Helen Keller

Your muse may be a song, a story, a sketch or a shade. Any one of these things can act as the 'on' switch for that little light bulb in your heart.

Cherish things that catch your eye and captivate you. Your choices are as unique as you.

'Do not quench your inspiration and imagination.'

Vincent Van Gogh

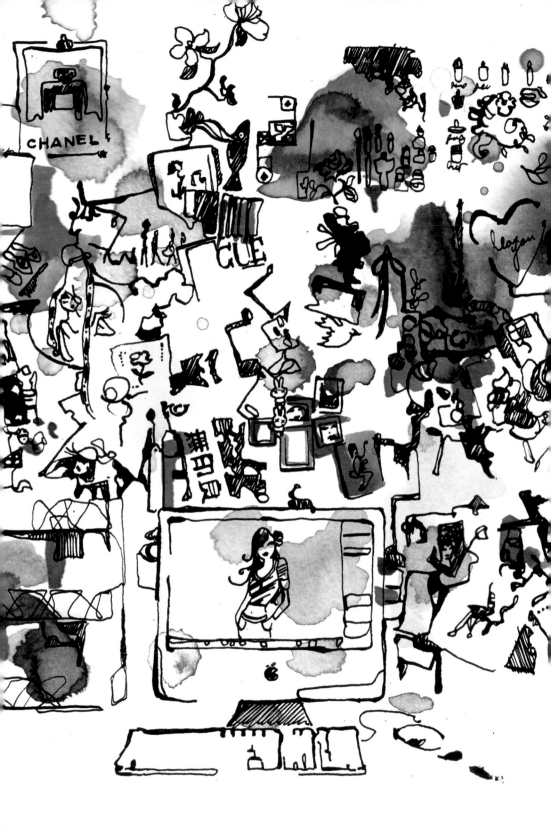

Pinboards, Paris and perfume

Pinboards are my way of reminding me of the trail I have taken. They are simply the most beautiful form of communication without words.

My pinboards embody many of my memories at a glance: a touchable, tactile album of imagination.

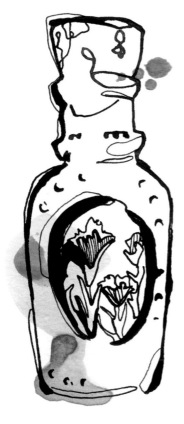
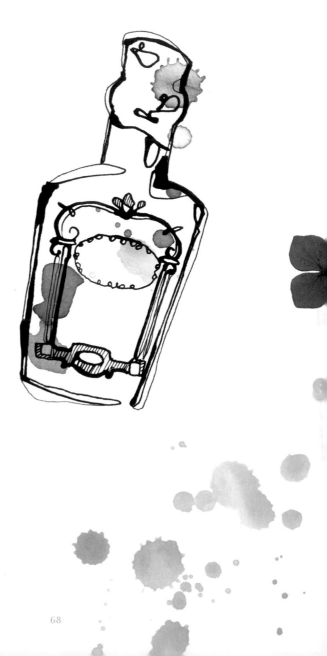

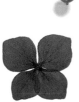

They showcase moments in time captured and hung like art from the heart. I collect everything and anything because I have loved it at some point. Even if I question a particular collection later, I know that it's inspired me before and can do so again.

I'm a bowerbird of all things beautiful, whether it be labels, colour swatches, ribbons, buttons, photos, stickers, postcards, food labels, fabric, origami paper, frames, jewellery, doilies, little cushions, confectionary wrappers, magazine pages, chocolate boxes, hairpins, swing tags, shopping bags or gallery invitations.

Alone they may just hum, but together on my pinboard, they simply sing!

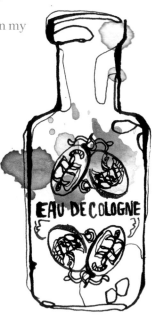

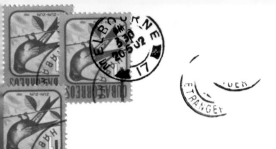

Strange as it may seem, I collect business cards. Not so much for the information but for what they remind me of and the way they look. It could be from a restaurant I love, a great innovative company, a quirky designer or a beautifully charming shop. Packaging, labels and swing tags have the same allure. They marry great graphics with clever delivery to catch our attention in an instant and set the tone for the product within.

We are bombarded with subliminal graphic messages throughout every day, and that is why I am so appreciative of the clever, quirky ones that really do it well and stand out from the rest.

Ribbons: What is it about these bands of coloured cloth in satin or silk?

Doilies: A paper-thin touch of the past made contemporary.

Buttons: Bright and beautiful, fragile and fine. Buttons make a statement in such a simple form.

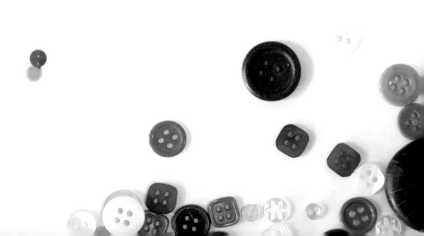

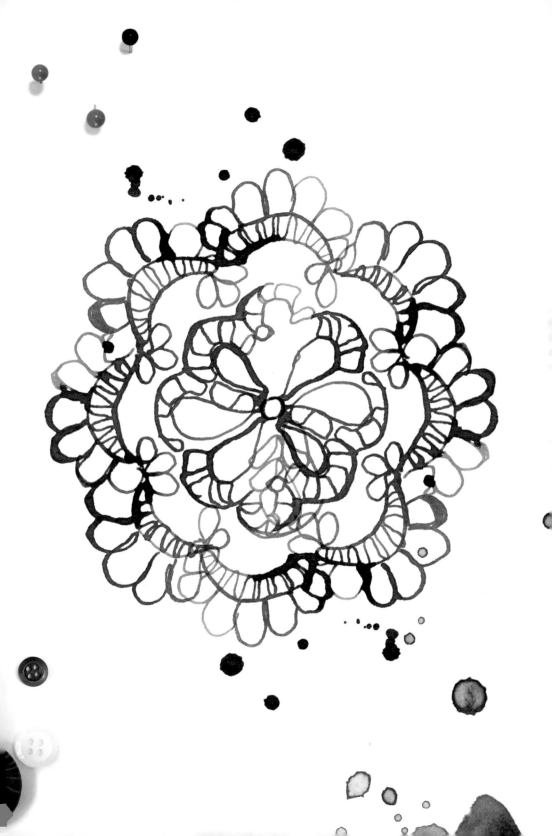

Paris

J'adore Paris. Every time I visit my favourite city,
I am in my element. The streets are beautiful, even
the plan of the city is enchanting. You can feel
the history in the art, music, poetry and fashion.
Buildings don't scrape the sky, they have their
own sense of place, full of architectural wisdom.
Everywhere you turn in Paris you see a set of
French doors opening into a private courtyard.
The city exudes heritage, romance and charm.

What I love most about Paris is the innate style of
Parisians which sets them apart. Not only in their
dress sense, but in the way they approach their
lives. Even a simple meal is a celebration.

The French find poetry in everyday life.

BY AIR MAIL
PAR AVION

'They have the ability to mix
the most random elements and
make them appear natural.
Very few can duplicate it.
It's unpredictable and I often
wish I could bottle it.'

My French Life,
Vicki Archer

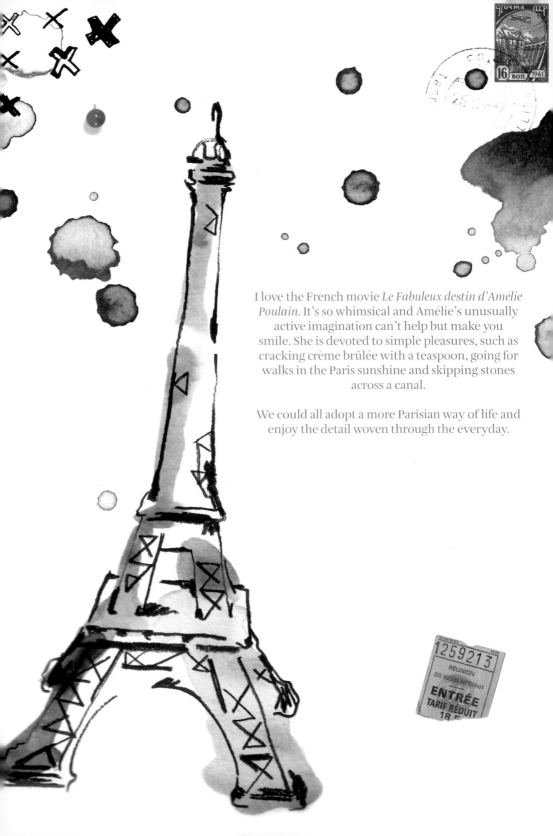

I love the French movie *Le Fabuleux destin d'Amélie Poulain*. It's so whimsical and Amélie's unusually active imagination can't help but make you smile. She is devoted to simple pleasures, such as cracking crème brûlée with a teaspoon, going for walks in the Paris sunshine and skipping stones across a canal.

We could all adopt a more Parisian way of life and enjoy the detail woven through the everyday.

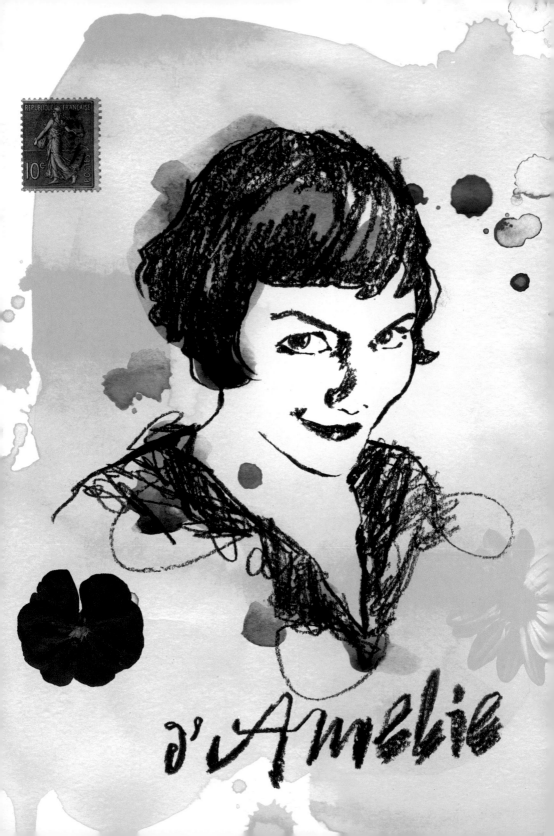

d'Amelie

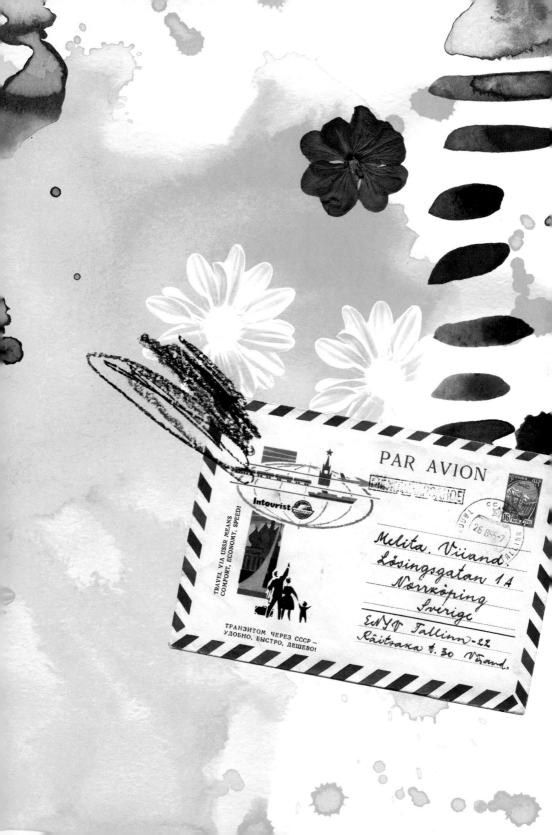

PAR AVION

ЗАКАЗНОЕ

Intourist

TRAVEL VIA USSR MEANS
COMFORT, ECONOMY, SPEED!

ТРАНЗИТОМ ЧЕРЕЗ СССР —
УДОБНО, БЫСТРО, ДЕШЕВО!

16 КОП

28.8.55-7

Melita. Viiand.
Lösingsgatan 14
Norrköping
Sverige
ENYF Tallinn-22
Räütsaka t. 30 Viiand.

Perfume

Perfume is the exclamation mark on the statement you are making. It's the magical finishing touch!

Just remember, marketing doesn't maketh the magical scent! I could never judge a perfume by its advertising. This is not a relationship that can be forged by a photograph. You have to experience a scent to really fall in love with it.

A fragrance is like a love affair; each time you invite that scent onto your skin, it forges your identity and leaves you feeling elegant, feminine and complete.

I buy perfumes for both the bouquet and the bottle. I love to collect perfume bottles; they are my glass menageries of romance and intrigue. An essential indulgence available to every woman.

'It is the unseen, unforgettable, ultimate accessory of fashion that heralds your arrival and prolongs your departure.'

Coco Chanel

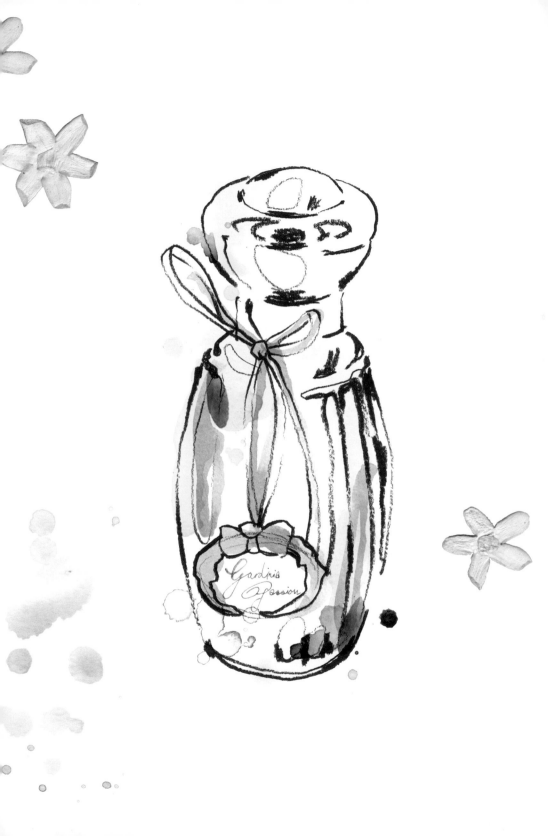

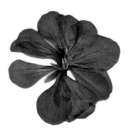

You never have to be loyal to one scent. Play the field of fragrances, and choose your armour to suit your mood. I have had various perfume stages throughout my life and each perfume marks the person I was at that time.

My first perfume as a teenager was Cacharel Anais Anais. I was captivated by the gorgeous floral packaging and I still love the sentiment of this fragrance.

I then moved on to Chloe, which my mum introduced me to. I later named my first daughter after this perfume and have a full set of oversized original Chloe bottles on display in her bedroom.

In my late teens I moved on to some pretty serious stuff from the big perfume houses. Now those scents give me a headache just thinking about them! Clearly I was making an overpowering statement during a time when I was breaking out and finding my feet.

Calvin Klein calmed me down in my twenties when Eternity and CK One came along. These lighter, fresher fragrances reflected an ease and subtle confidence in my life.

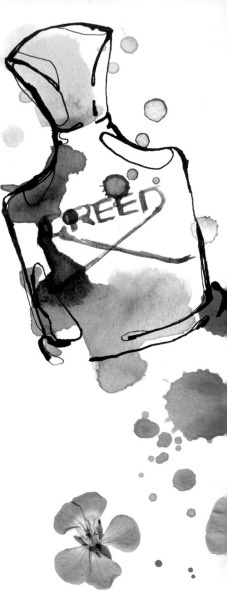

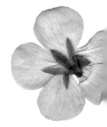

In my mid twenties, during a trip to Paris,
I discovered Annick Goutal Gardenia Passion.
It opened a new world of scent to me and I have
never looked back. Gardenia Passion has perfectly
captured the seduction of blossoming gardenias.

A decade on I still wear Gardenia Passion but now
I love to mix it up with other scents including:

Creed Spring Flower is rumoured to have been
originally designed for Audrey Hepburn. Vibrant
fresh green notes combine with succulent fruits
over a floral heart of jasmine and rose.

Frederic Malle makes perfumes without
compromise. He personally recommended Lys
Méditerranée to me and said I would never forget
him. He was right. Lys Méditerranée is a heady
blend that pays tribute to the opulent scent of
ginger lily. Its fresh accent definitely leaves an
impression.

Annick Goutal Le Jasmin: this perfume makes me
think of spring. It is a fresh and sparkling scent
with a hint of spicy ginger.

Santa Maria Novella Mughetto: Mughetto
translated from Italian is lily of the valley ...
what more do I need to say? I also love this scent
because it reminds me of a very good friend.

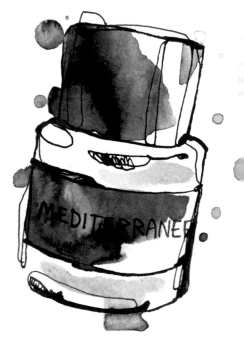

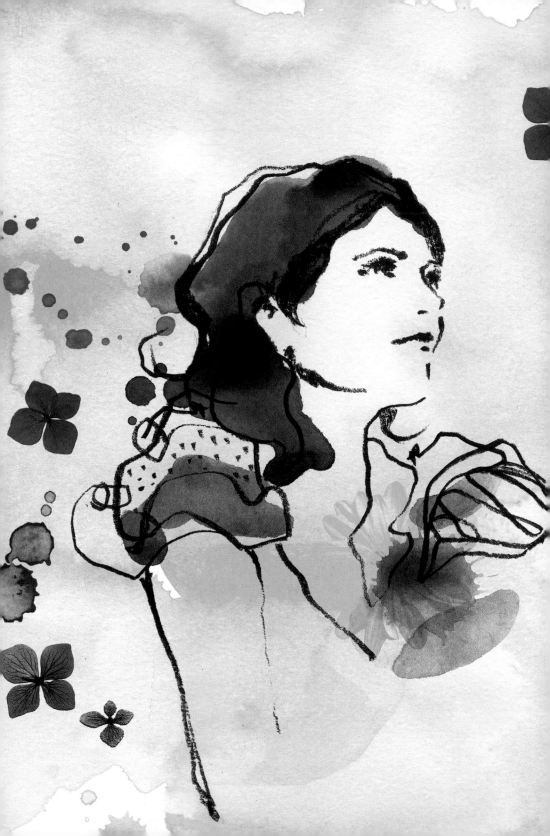

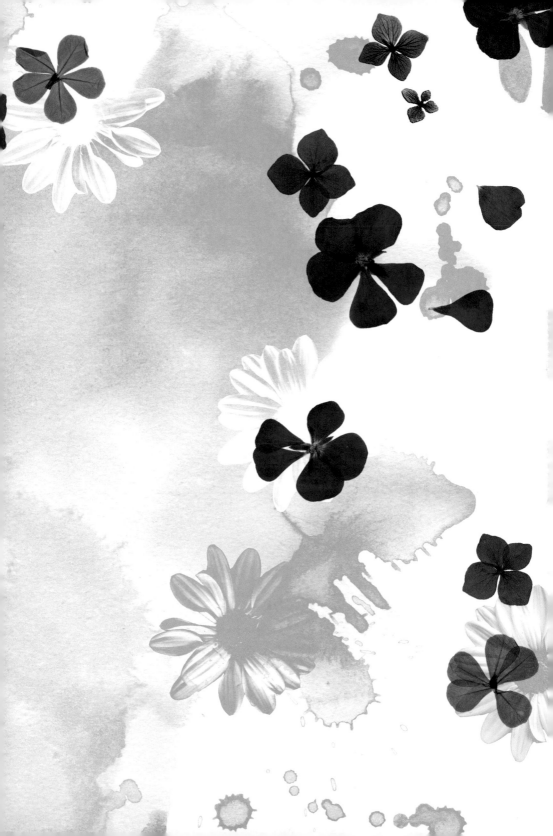

Collect and create

Collecting without rhyme or reason is a joy. Surround yourself with the things you love. Having the things I love around me has always acted as a catalyst for my next creation.

Follow your heart, follow your interests. Pursue what you adore.

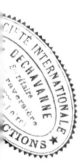

Notebooks

There is nothing more inviting than a clean, crisp, new page. The humble notebook exudes elegance and old-fashioned charm in a high-tech world.

Writing is such a feminine notion: sitting down to a notebook and a pen and taking the time to communicate with yourself, or others.

I've always got several notebooks on the go for jotting down something funny the kids might say or a memory I don't want to forget. It's a way to capture the freshness of the moment for the future.

Handwriting and notebooks give words the life typing deprives them of. A personality appears in every curve and loop.

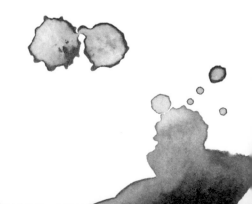

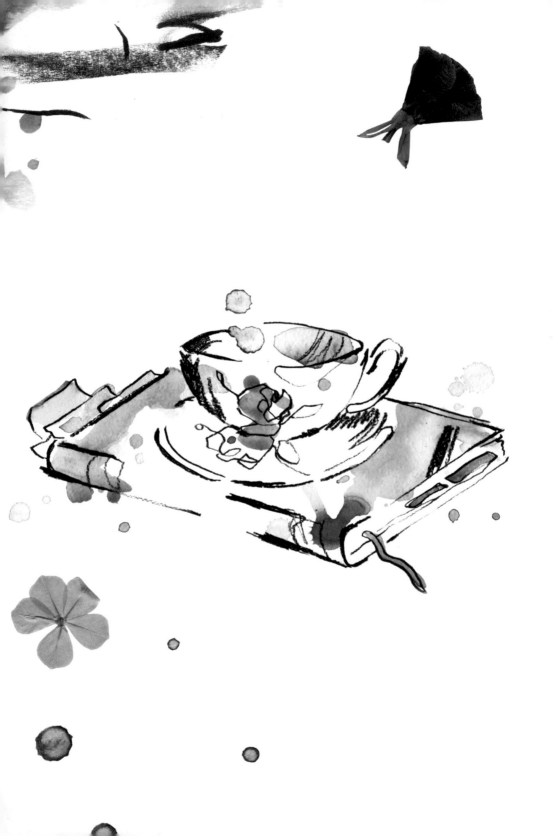

MIRKA MORA

The Complete DMC Encyclopedia of Needlework

A GARDENER'S LOG

FASHIONS IN MAKUP

Color Source Book

TEXTILE DESIGNS

THE GARDEN BOOK

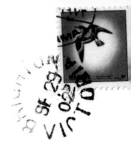

Books

Books are an infinite source of inspiration. Stacked a-clutter or filed in line, books add soul to your home, their spines facing us, their stories secret whispers amongst themselves.

The true beauty of a book is that it contains no strangers, just friends you haven't got to know yet. And over the years you can return and cast an eye across their cover, run a finger over their words, and these old friends will awaken and provide a new lesson every time.

I love collecting books about cosmetics, colour, embroidery, crochet, lace, design and textiles. But most of all I love autobiographies and reading about other people's incredibly interesting lives.

When a friend I trust refers a book, I will go to the ends of the earth to get it. That mission to find it makes devouring that book so much sweeter.

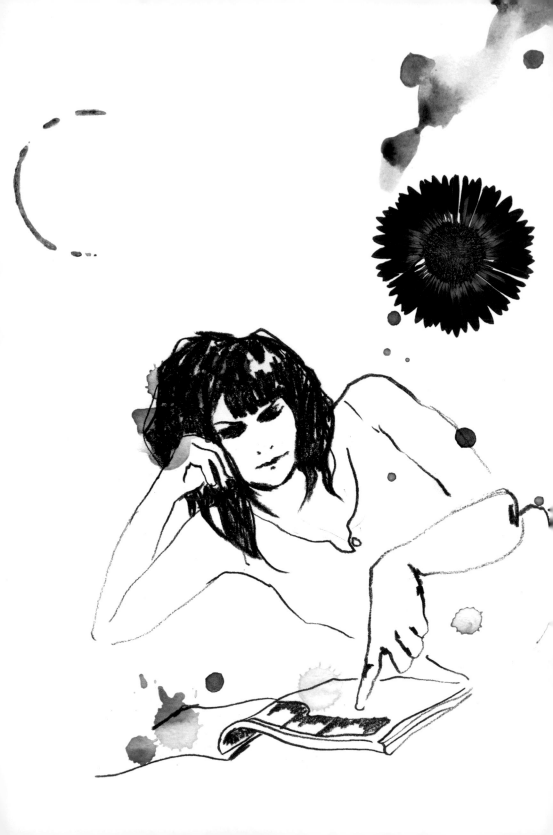

Magazines

If a book is a marriage, then a magazine is more
of a fling.

From a fashion point of view, magazines represent
a moment in time waiting to be revisited.
Magazines keep pace with the heartbeat of now.
When now becomes then, flicking through the
pages takes you back. They are less a snapshot of
style, as they are pieces of a puzzle that cumulate
in a movement, a trend, or an iconic image.

I have always found magazines irresistible. I have
at least two decades' worth that I simply can't part
with! They might be more disposable than books,
but magazines are still impossible to throw away.
For once they're gone, they're gone forever.

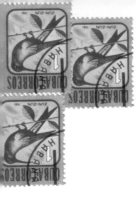

DIY

The joy of painting, knitting, crocheting, embroidery, sewing or beading can allow respite for a moment and an alternative to the modern-day speed of technology.

It becomes an obsession with no rehab, but a safe and lovely obsession no less. So revel in it.

'Something you create yourself
is the best kind of present.'

Jacqueline Kennedy Onassis

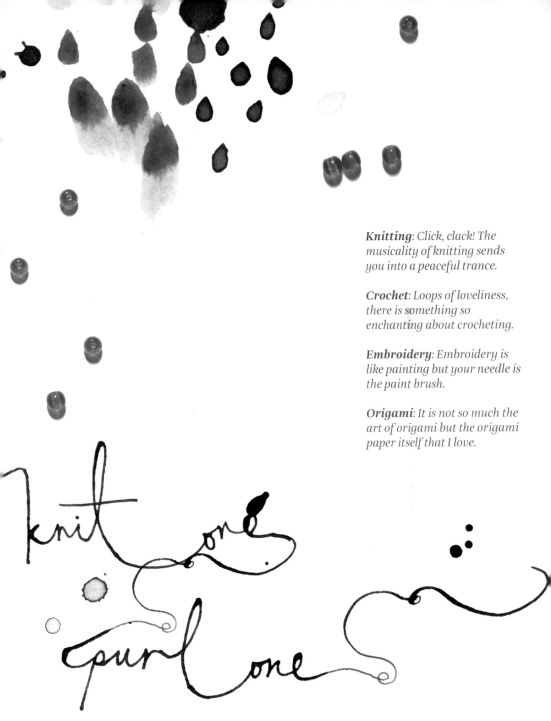

Knitting: Click, clack! The musicality of knitting sends you into a peaceful trance.

Crochet: Loops of loveliness, there is something so enchanting about crocheting.

Embroidery: Embroidery is like painting but your needle is the paint brush.

Origami: It is not so much the art of origami but the origami paper itself that I love.

origami paper flowers

1. FOLD IN HALF

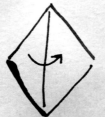

2. FOLD LEFT & RIGHT CORNERS TO MEET IN THE CENTRE

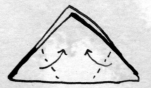

3. FOLD IN HALF

4. CUT FOLDED PAPER FOLLOWING IDEAS BELOW AND UNFOLD.

A.

B.

C.

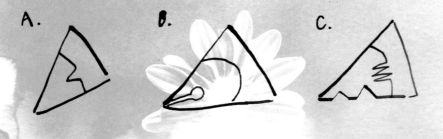

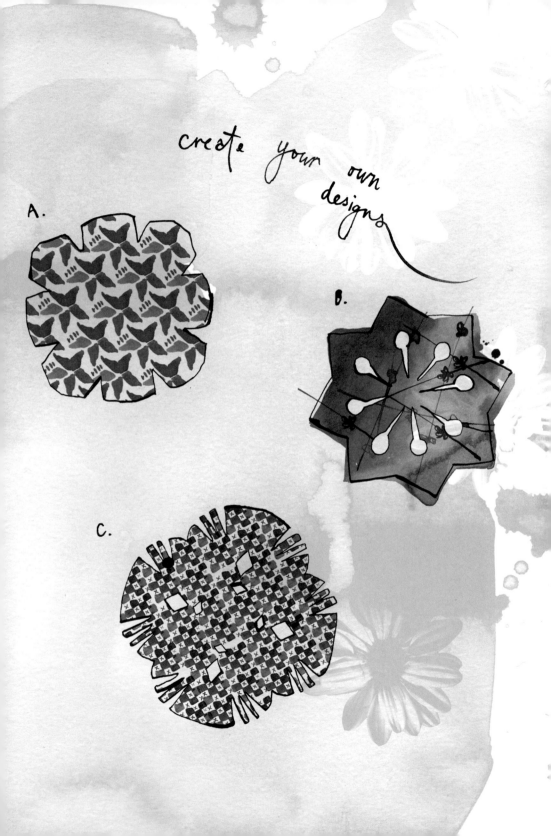

create your own
designs

A.

B.

C.

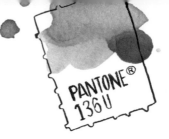

PANTONE® 136U

Colour

Colour motivates me to create. It is like a visual embrace. I'm crazy about it; from Pantone chips and embroidery swatches to paint charts and Derwent pencils. Dipping into pots of watercolour and tubes of paint gives me so much direction for my cosmetics.

PANTONE® 179U

ANTONE® 31U

PANTONE® 213U

PANTONE® 272U

PANTONE® 072U

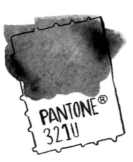

PANTONE® 321U

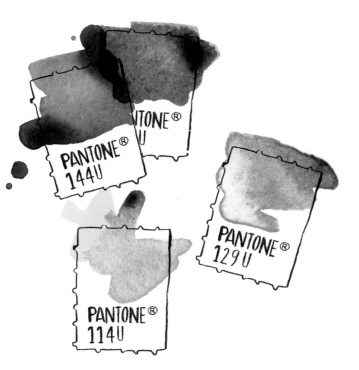

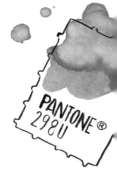

Les goûts et les couleurs ne se discutent pas.
Taste and colour one does not discuss.
French saying

I love this French saying. It is hard to translate
but to me it means that something like colour is
such a personal thing that it can't be questioned.
What a colour means to me is not the same
as what it means to you. Colour is a personal
intimate experience. Everybody has their own
special colour.

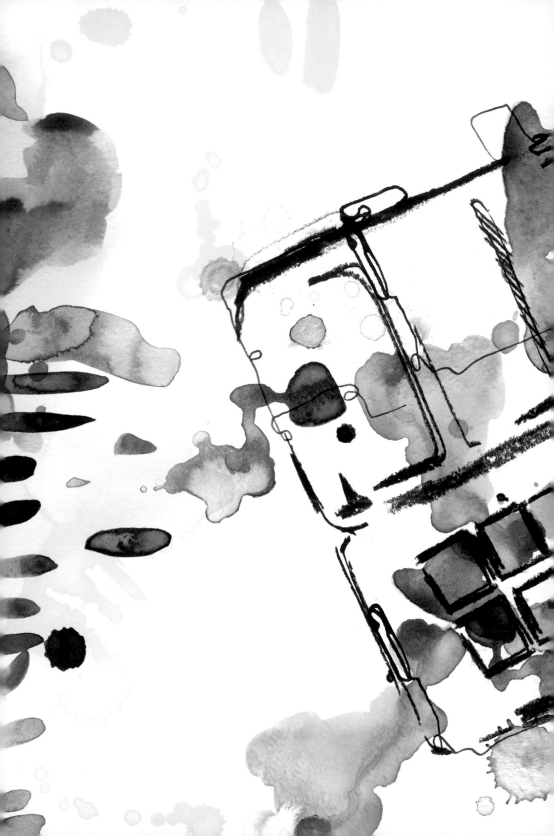

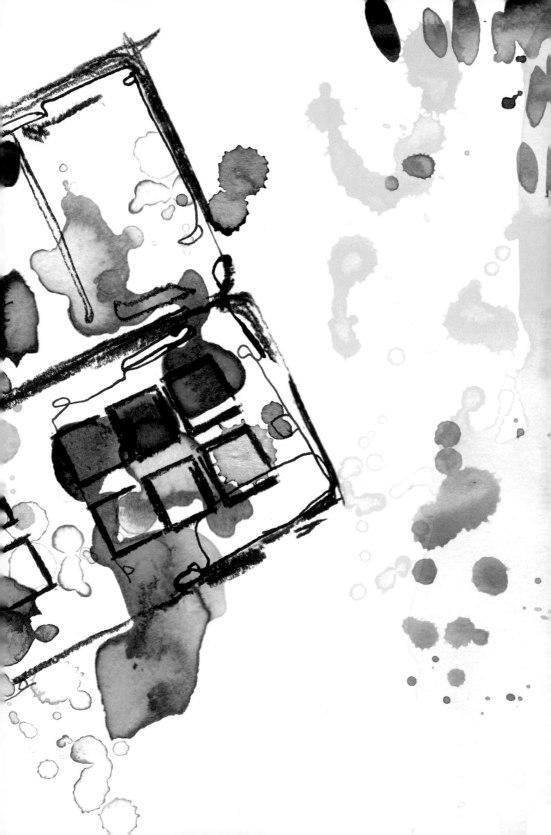

The beauty in nature

As a very visual person, I am often overwhelmed by the simple pleasure I get from the form, colour and texture of the flowers, leaves and trees right outside my door. The beauty of nature is so effortless.

One who plants a garden
plants happiness.

Proverb

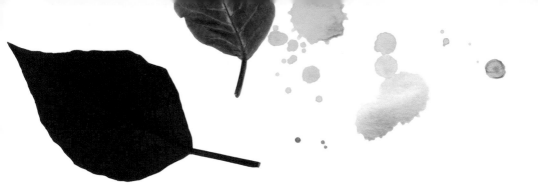

Gardens

Gardening grows the soul, for in a garden life ends
simply to begin again.

Experience the scent of spring, the change of
autumn, the chill of winter and the heat of
summer as the colours, aromas and textures shift
with each season.

I chose the plants for my garden at home based
on their perfume, their colour and the fruits and
flowers they yield. I get great joy from my garden
and relish time enjoying its beauty and evolution.

I particularly love Edna Walling gardens. They
are undulating, enchanted, eclectic, wild and
unpredictable.

Even so, I often think that designing gardens is
something of a misnomer. How can you wrangle
and tame something that has a mind of its own
into your vision? Flowers should be encouraged
to take on their own personalities. Like a sea of
children, let them grow in their own directions,
chasing their own sunshine and establishing
themselves as unique and beautiful beings to be
cherished independently.

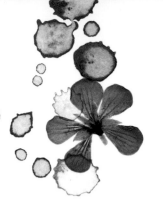
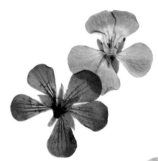

Flowers

Flowers are the pinnacle of feel-good gifts. Always making people feel better and happier, flowers are sunshine to the soul. So, bring Mother Nature's show-and-tell inside.

White flowers are the most fragrant and the heart and soul of perfumery: gardenia, freesia, jasmine, hyacinth, daphne, tuberose, and lily of the valley.

My favourite flower of all is the peony rose. I love the delicacy of their densely packed petals, and the clustered chaos makes the imperfections of their blossoms even more perfect. Peony roses bloom around my birthday—and for such a short time—so their 'blink and you'll miss us' quality makes them all the more ethereal, unattainable and appreciated. They are nature's birthday gift to me!

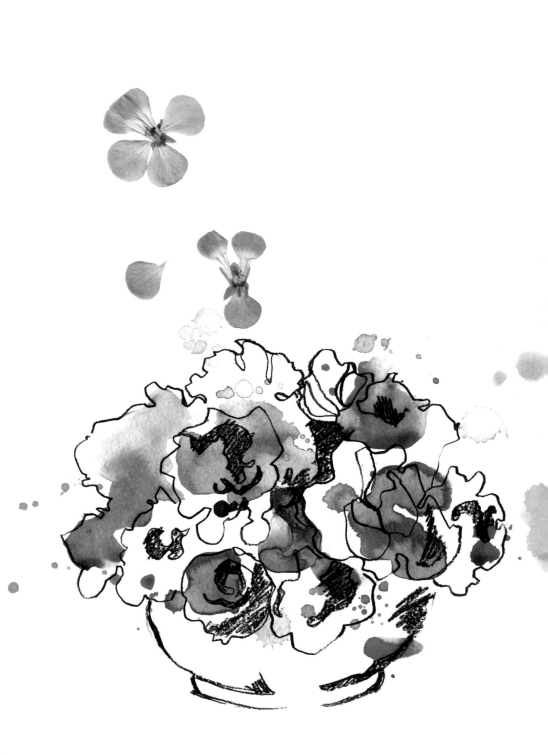

'Flowers are love's truest
language.'

Park Benjamin

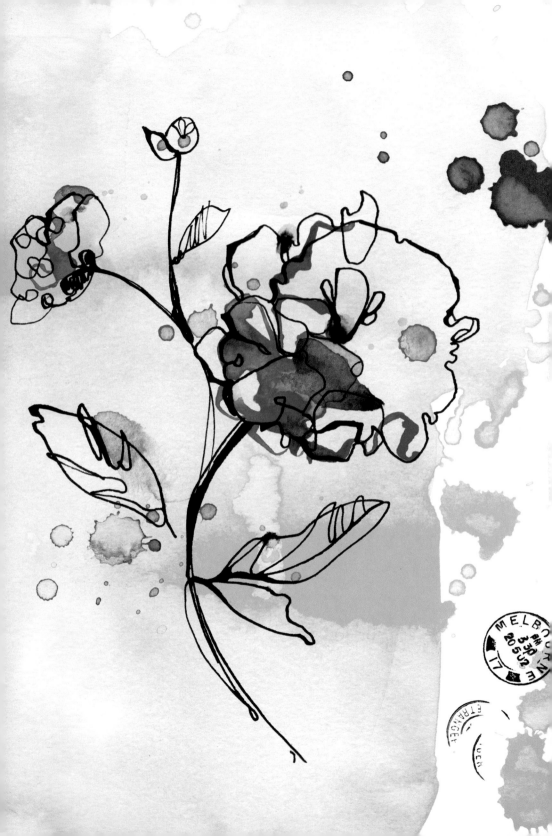

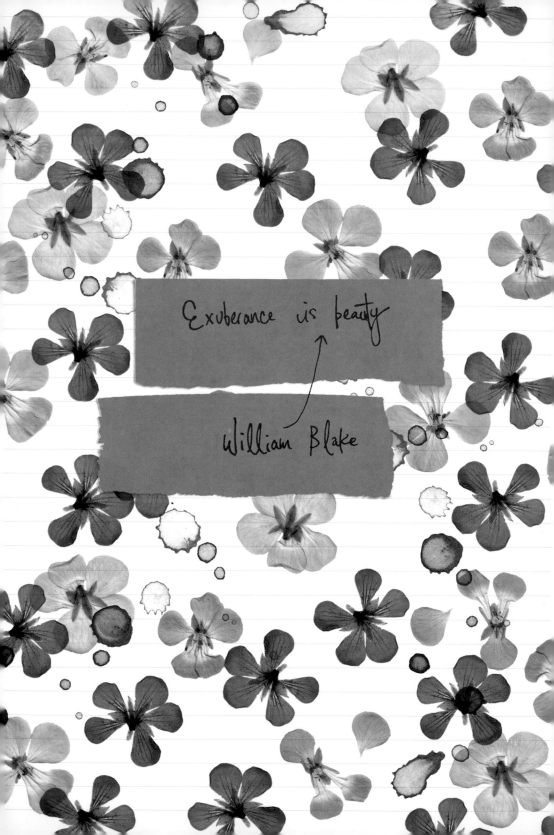

Exuberance is beauty

William Blake

Conclusion

I love living life to the fullest and soaking up everything. Follow your dreams, let your heart guide you and surround yourself with people you love and who inspire you. Be passionate and look after yourself.

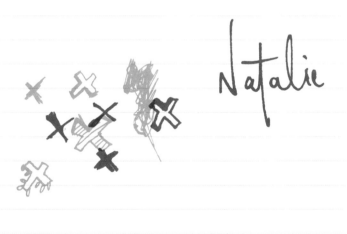

Natalie

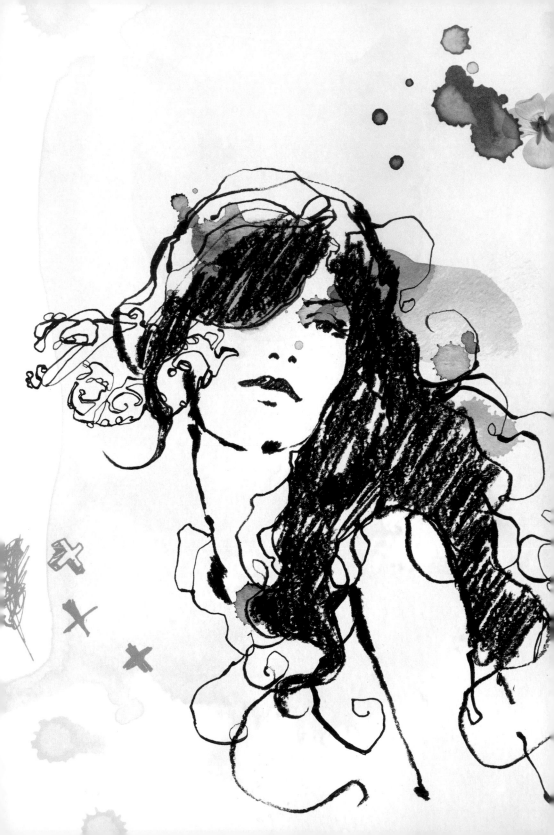

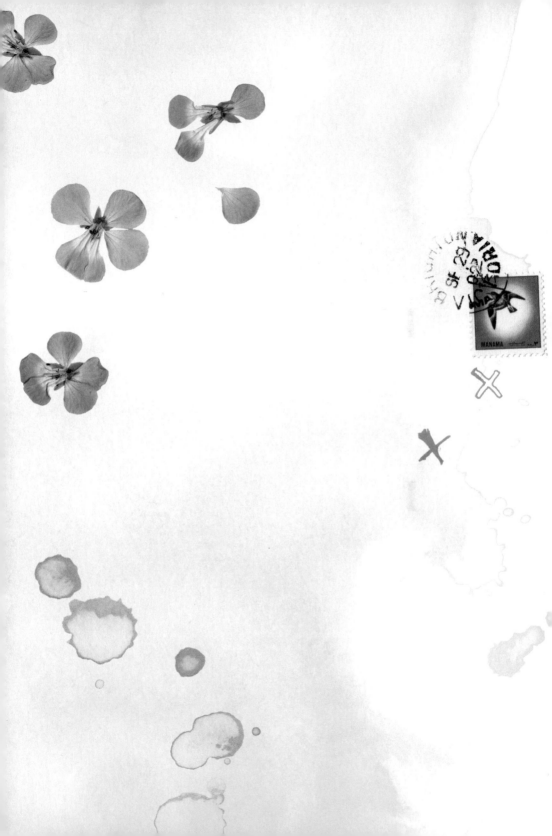

Acknowledgements

Emma-Charlotte Bangay, thank you for sharing this journey with me and for taking on such a huge challenge. I appreciate your endless enthusiasm and your sensitivity to ensure each word represented my true sentiment.

Thank you to Elise Garland for so many things; without your initial excitement for the opportunity to write a book, this project would never have eventuated. Thank you also for your incredible publicity efforts, continued support and, most of all, our friendship.

Catherine Milne, from Allen and Unwin, thank you for planting the seed for *Beauty in Bloom* and allowing it to blossom in its own unique way. Your patience, authenticity and guidance through every stage are greatly appreciated.

Brian Hamersfeld, my incredible husband. Without your infectious spirit and encouragement I would never have had the guts to start my own business in the first place. You fill our lives with so much fun and you continue to inspire me and allow me to follow my passions. I love you.

To my gorgeous children: Chloe, Amber and Zac, you fill me up with joy and happiness everyday. And to Justin, you are always with me. I am bursting with love for all of you.

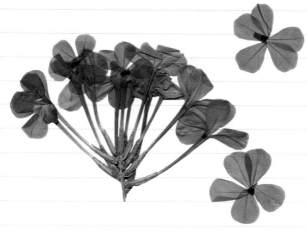

To my mum, dad, brother and sister. I couldn't do half of what I do without your love and support. Thank you for being there in my highs and lows.

Melissa Murphy. Thank you for loving our children and for allowing me to balance work and motherhood. You are amazing.

Thank you to the whole Bloom team for your day-to-day support and, in particular, Clare Hillier and Evie Smith for your suggestions, ideas and genuine joy through each stage of this book.

Rebecca Wetzler. Thank you for your elegant illustrations, they are so full of passion and life. I cannot believe how effortlessly you turned each idea into the perfect image. You are such a gifted illustrator.

Thank you to Ryan Guppy, who brought my vision for this book to life and much, much more. I am full of admiration for your incredible design eye, appreciation for typography and colour, empathy for illustration and pattern and your ability to make clutter feel organised and balanced. It was a pleasure to work with you.

First published in the UK in 2009 by
Apple Press
7 Greenland Street
London NW1 0ND
United Kingdom
www.apple-press.com

First published in Australia in 2008 by
Allen & Unwin
83 Alexander Street
Crows Nest NSW 2065
Australia
Phone: (61 2) 8425 0100
Fax: (61 2) 9906 2218
Email: info@allenandunwin.com
Web: www.allenandunwin.com

Aesthetics--Philosophy

111.85

ISBN 978 1 84543 326 0

Design by 21-19 (www.21-19.com)
Illustrations by Rebecca Wetzler
Printed in China by Everbest Printing Co., Ltd

www.bloomcosmetics.com

10 9 8 7 6 5 4 3 2 1

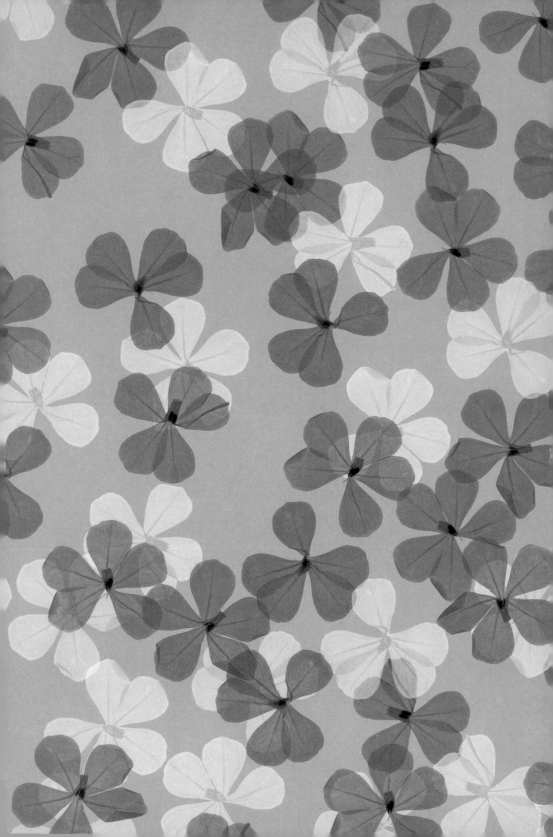